Building DEMS:

Keeping Depression, Anxiety and Stress at Bay

Dr Justin Peter

About the Author

Dr. Justin Peter (EdD) is a trainer, therapist and coach for those who seek meaning and purpose in their lives, relationships and work. He believes that change and empowerment start from the inside out – beginning with an understanding of our innate personalities, emotions and life experiences. He is a certified behavioural consultant and practitioner in Reality Therapy. His research interests include psychological types and the learning brain. In his free time, Justin enjoys watching Netflix and practices *shinrin-yoku*.

Readers with questions or engagement requests can email him at: approach.justin@gmail.com

Is this book for you?

Wondering if you should read this book? Go through the following items and check those that often or sometimes describe your current situation.

- I overthink about many things.

- I battle with low moods.

- I am experiencing stress and burnout.

- I have difficulties managing my work and/or relationships.

- My mind is occupied with anxieties and worries.

- I have trouble relaxing and winding down.

- Sleep problems are affecting my physical, mental and emotional health.

- My thought life is affecting my real life.

- I don't have the motivation, desire or energy to get out and about.

- I would like additional help in improving my mental and emotional well-being apart from therapy and medication.

If some of these statements apply to you, you might benefit from the principles and techniques offered in the pages of this book. Read on to find out how you can implement DEMS in your life and enhance your personal well-being.

Contents

1
Introduction

Dwelling on problems will not help us overcome them, because we will be unable to see the answer we need. Solutions are found, on the other hand, when we see things in a new and fresh way.

Richard Carlson

In 2009, I embarked on a three-day kayaking trip around Cheow Lan Lake in Khao Sok National Park, Thailand. Touted as one of the most beautiful places in the country, the sprawling lake was surrounded by magnificent limestone cliffs and dense forests that are home to elephants, tigers, tapirs and monkeys. Looking down from my kayak, a dreamlike scene greeted me – a landscape of trees and vegetation fully submerged under the tranquil waters. And they have been hidden there for decades.

My guide explained that I was actually kayaking above what was once the canopy of a rainforest in a valley. Cheow Lan Lake was formed as a result of building the Ratchaprapa Dam in 1982. Taking a year for the valley to be filled with water, the hydroelectric dam subsequently paved the way for irrigation, flood control and power generation.

All around the world, dams perform important roles. They help to store floodwaters during rainstorms, and release them in a controlled manner to the rivers below or channel them for other uses. Some dams also trap debris while allowing clear water to pass through.

While strong and effective dams benefit the townsfolk and the surrounding regions, a burst dam can unleash unparalleled damage. Throughout history, the sudden release of massive volumes of water from the dam failures have been known to cause human causalities, wipe out physical properties and harm the natural environment.

Of course, this book is not about these physical dams. I use dams as an analogy to demonstrate the importance of upkeeping our personal well-being and mental fortitude so that we are not overwhelmed by the troubled waters of depression, anxiety and stress. I term this state of being mentally and emotionally overwhelmed as *psychological flooding*.

Psychological Flooding

Depression, anxiety and stress are no strangers in today's world. In fact, they have been on the rise in recent decades. School counsellors are seeing an increasing number of students buckling under the demands of academia, self-image and peer pressure. In offices all over, employers and employees alike are struggling with work-related stresses and a decline in work-life balance. Breakdowns in marriages and family systems are also contributing towards mental and emotional health concerns.

In picking up this book, you might be looking for some help to cope with a certain life issue that seems overwhelming. Or perhaps you might know someone who could benefit from this resource. It is worthwhile noting that it is not the intent of this book to help you diagnose depression, anxiety or stress, although I will very briefly touch on these issues to provide some context for psychological flooding. If you haven't already done so, you are encouraged to seek professional help for a clinical understanding of what you might be experiencing.

Depression

Carl, a company executive in his forties, was going through a rough patch in his marriage. While talks about divorce were on the table, Carl was not looking forward to be separated from his wife. He felt that the marriage could be salvaged. Thus, he tried ways and means to mend the relationship. While initially hopeful, months of trying were met with repeated disappointments and rejections. By the time Carl came to my office, he was downtrodden and riddled with self-blame. Constant thoughts about how sad and terrible life was contributed towards psychological flooding in his mind. He started to interpret things around him negatively. Soon, Carl lost the motivation to exercise or socialise, and sunk deeper into despair.

Truth be told, no one can be happy all the time. There's bound to be bumps in the road. And sometimes, sadness can be an appropriate response. We all experience this emotion at some point or another. Feelings of sadness can be a result of going through trigger events such as a loss or a difficult situation in life. Overtime, you may learn to manage our problems or accept the changes in your life. However, the sadness can sometimes become so overwhelming that it interferes with your everyday activities and normal functioning. Like Carl, your thoughts, emotions and behaviours may be dominated by a sense of profound sadness. And you are not able to cope as you used to. When sadness of this degree does not go away, you may be facing what is clinically known as depression.

Symptoms of depression may include:

- Persistent sadness and despair.

- Feelings of worthlessness or guilt.

- Loss of interest in activities previously enjoyed.

- Feeling tired or lethargic.

- Feeling agitated or restless.

- Difficulties sleeping or sleeping excessively.

- Decrease or increase in appetite and weight.

There're many reasons why you might be stuck in depression. Some people said that they just couldn't find it in themselves to accept the circumstances or flaws in their lives. Others are seeking some form external validation, such as success, love or wealth, before they can feel happy. I'm guessing your situation might be unique, with its own sets of challenges and complexities. Whichever the case, I hope that by gleaning the principles in this book and putting them into practice, you might find some relief.

Anxiety

Anxieties can take many forms. For example, performance anxiety, social anxiety or specific fears or phobias. If you think about it, anxieties can keep you safe and help you better manage certain risks or harm. While it is normal to feel anxious every once in a while, severe anxiety can adversely affect a person's daily functioning – especially when you become a prisoner to your thoughts. This could come in the form of excessive worrying, analysing or brooding over the worst-case scenarios. I'll use the term "rumination" to refer to these forms of overthinking.

Pam described her experience of psychological flooding as a "hurricane" that revolved non-stop around concerns about her health. She developed a heightened sense of alertness, and linked any discomfort in her body to diseases that she perceived she might be having. Worries raced around in Pam's mind, and one thing led to another. She thought her headaches were caused by brain cancer, and a shortness-of-breath an impending heart attack. Minor symptoms would be blown out of proportion. Doctors gave Pam a clean bill of health, but referred her for help with her anxieties.

For others, anxieties can revolve around things such as health, relationships, finances, job responsibilities, socialising or being in certain places or situations. Anxieties can also shift from one thing to another over time and age. Whichever form your anxious rumination takes, it can consume enormous amounts of time and energy. Rumination can become a loop – the more you submerse in it, the harder it is to snap out of it. The resulting despair and stress often take a toll on your mental and emotional well-being.

Apart from the excessive worrying which Pam faced, anxiety may also be accompanied by symptoms such as:

- Difficulty concentrating

- Indecisiveness

- Lethargy

- Nervousness

- Faster heartbeats

- Head discomfort
- Churning or fluttering stomach
- Cold feet and hands
- Hand trembles
- Dry mouth
- Panic attacks

In Cognitive Behavioural Therapy (CBT), there is an adage that goes: You **feel** the way you **think**. From this view, there's a good chance that your rumination is contributing to your anxiety and low moods rather than the circumstances of your life. As you go through this book, you will better grasp the nature of your thoughts, and learn to relate to them differently.

Stress

Stress can be seen as our body's way of responding to threats or demands. These demands could be imposed on us by ourselves or by others. We could also impose demands on others, and feel stressed when things are not done properly. Factors such as unrealistic expectations, uncertainties and changes can contribute towards stress. Of the different stress triggers, work is steadily becoming one of the biggest sources of stress in today's modern society.

When his company was going through a re-structuring process, Keith got worried about his job security. Thoughts about becoming unemployed, and remaining unemployed, flooded his mind. Being the sole bread-winner of his young family, he could not afford to go without an income. Furthermore, he had grown to love the work he was doing. Keith eventually remained in the company, albeit with an increased workload – he was given additional duties which were previously managed by colleagues who had left. Determined not to drop the ball, Keith devoted more time and energy at work. Sleep and leisure became a luxury. In the little time he had with his family, his mind was constantly stressed about work. On the verge of a burnout, Keith knew he had to start making changes to his hectic lifestyle.

Stress can be positive or negative, depending on the situation. Moderately stressful events can be good for us. They keep our brains more alert, making us perform better. Our brains respond by adapting and growing. On the other hand, negative stress, like what Keith was experiencing, can make us overwhelmed and distressed, leading to health problems and exhaustion.

Stressful situations are part and parcel of life. While external events can cause us stress, the stress can be induced by our own mental perception of those events. Thus, the same event experienced by different persons can result in very different responses. For example, when tasked to make a public presentation, one who sees it as a growth opportunity might spend extra time preparing and rehearsing, while another who perceives it as fearful or embarrassing might be frozen with distress. It becomes harmful when people turn to unhealthy behaviours or substances to relief stress.

The DEMS Approach to Personal Well-being

Stressors and triggers of various nature can be very much present in our lives. Without a healthy level of mind, you may find yourself caving under these trigger events and being psychologically flooded. Coming back to the analogy of dams – just like how a burst dam can cause flooding and harm, psychological flooding can impair your ability to manage your thoughts and emotions. As Carl, Pam and Keith have experienced, you may feel like things are spiralling beyond control.

By contrast, a strong dam is akin to having a healthy personal well-being. The ability to manage your physical, mental and emotional health in your daily living can help to prevent psychological flooding when things don't seem to go your way. To help you achieve that, I will be sharing with you about DEMS – an approach which I have put together to help my clients in their journey towards personal wellness.

"DEMS" is the acronym of the four key elements of the approach, namely:

Diet – **Chapter 2** touches on the importance of having balanced and regular meals, and making changes to your diet to help your brain and body function more effectively. This includes omega-3 fatty acids and ample hydration.

Engaging activities – In **Chapter 3**, you will learn about the positive impact that engaging activities can have on your mind. Being mentally engaged by work, exercise and leisure activities boosts your personal well-being.

Mindfulness – **Chapter 4** provides an introduction to mindfulness and recommends certain mindfulness practices to incorporate in your daily routine, which can help you curb rumination and stay centered.

Sleep – The benefits of having ample rest will be talked about in **Chapter 5**. If you are struggling with insomnia, look out for the section on managing your sleep worries with mindfulness.

Each of these four elements is research-informed and evidence-based. Practitioners worldwide have used one or more of these components in advancing personal wellness. The DEMS approach presented in this book combines these four components into an integrated plan to help you cope with depression, manage anxiety and reduce stress. **Chapter 6** suggests a format where you can tie up these four components together and keep track your progress.

Bear in mind, though, that the DEMS approach is not a quick-fix. Think of it as more of a lifestyle – building and implementing your personalised DEMS plan consistently during peaceful times can cushion the negative impact of the not-so-peaceful times.

How DEMS Came About

Over the years, I saw an increasing number of clients who were struggling with depression, anxiety as well as stress arising from work and personal life. Counselling techniques such as CBT and Reality Therapy, which I was trained in, formed the core of my helping model during my early years as a practitioner. In the last decade, I began researching for more ways to support my clients apart from the offer of counselling or coaching, which some would term as "talk therapy". While talk therapy was helpful in allowing my clients to process their thoughts and perspectives, I wanted a holistic treatment approach which clients could implement in their everyday lives –

simple changes to their lifestyle which they could execute on their own (or with a little help).

My research led me to the works of practitioners who explored the benefits of making certain lifestyle adjustments that could enhance one's mental and emotional well-being. Most notably, Dr Stephen Ilardi (2010) found that the Therapeutic Lifestyle Change (TLC) method produced promising results in treating depression. The TLC is a six-step method that includes Omega-3 fatty acids supplements, anti-rumination strategies, exercise, light exposure, social support and sleep hygiene. This natural method posed success rates that are comparable to the use of medication.

More recently, in the field of personal development and executive coaching, Sara Milne Rowe (2018) – a leading performance coach in the UK – developed the SHED method to help her clients achieve "confidence, calm and success". The set of mind-management techniques comprise of sleep, hydration, exercise and diet.

I was intrigued by TLC's approach in managing depression without medication. The SHED method has some similar elements, but aimed at performance coaching. For me, this meant that these elements can contribute towards therapeutic, preventive and developmental outcomes. Inspired, I integrated these elements with principles of Reality Therapy and mindfulness to form the DEMS approach for my own clients who were going through challenging and difficult times in their lives.

This book you are holding is not intended to be a heavy or lengthy thesis on managing ones' personal well-being. In contrast, it is designed to be a practical guide to facilitate implementation of the DEMS approach. I also avoid the use of complicated jargons. It was originally intended to serve as an accompaniment to the coaching sessions for my clients. That is, until one of them mooted the idea of sharing it with a wider audience who could benefit from its principles. As you read through this book, I hope that you, too, will find it an easy read and helpful for your particular context.

On Changing Your Thoughts – Not Easy!

Remember the adage – *you feel the way you think*? I do agree, to a large extent, that issues such as depression, anxiety and stress are contributed by our thoughts. There is an intricate interaction among our thoughts, emotions and physiology that results in and amplifies these issues. For this reason, many models of psychotherapy (such as CBT) aim to help you to change or reframe your "negative thoughts" to positive or more balanced ones so that improved moods will follow. And this is where I deviate slightly.

If you are someone who can rather easily adopt positive thinking and reframe your negative beliefs, that's great! But if you have struggled with it, you're not alone. I know how difficult it can be to change our thoughts… even if we know they are "negative". If the achievement of your mental and emotional well-being is tied solely to your ability to reframe your thoughts, then it can be a steep uphill climb.

But all is not lost…

Here's the good news - change can begin with your actions. Yes, even small, baby steps can go a long way in improving your personal well-being. And actions can be easier to change compared to your thoughts.

Let me try to illustrate this with this simple *activity*, which I'll need your help with. Find a quiet place where you can be comfortably seated without distractions. The activity will take about a minute. Ready to go? Try your best to carry out the following instructions:

- First, stretch your left arm forward such that it is parallel with the ground.

- Slowly put your left arm down.

- Next, stretch your right arm forward such that it is parallel with the ground.

- Turn your right hand so that your palm is facing upwards.

- With your right arm still outstretched, imagine there's a green apple on your palm (you can close your eyes if it helps you to visualise better).

- Now, instead of a green apple, imagine a red apple on your palm.

- Next, imagine a big worm crawling out of the red apple.

- As you see the worm, you start to feel frightened.

- Then, you begin to sweat and tremble with fright.

- Activity complete! You can put your arm down now and open your eyes if they were closed.

Let's take some time to review what happened: Which instructions were easier to follow? Which were more challenging?

I've done this activity with many people during training and coaching sessions. All of them thought that the instructions to stretch their arms and turn their palms were the easiest to comply with. These instructions are to do with **actions**.

Many felt that imagining the apples and worm were the next easiest to do. However, for some people it was challenging to conjure these images in their minds. These instructions are to do with **thoughts**.

Finally, almost everyone had difficulties trying to "feel frightened" and to "sweat and tremble". These are to do with **emotions** and **physiology** respectively.

So, what does this tell us about the journey towards an improved mental and emotional health? Getting you to start by changing your physiology and emotions is going to be a challenge. It's like telling a friend in depression to "cheer up" and "don't be sad" – while it is done with good intent, it might not be the most helpful. Feelings and physiology are hard to change on their own. In comparison, cognitive methods like modifying or reframing beliefs are easier since they are to do with thoughts. But the path with least resistance, so to speak, is to work on making certain adjustments to your actions, habits and lifestyle.

Think of these components – actions, thoughts, emotions and physiology – as the four wheels of a car. The front wheels are actions and thoughts. When they change direction as a result of being steered, the back wheels, which are emotions and physiology, will eventually follow suit.

And this is what DEMS is about – getting you to take action by adjusting your diet, scheduling engaging activities, practising mindfulness and having ample sleep. And hopefully, like what many others have experienced, your moods will gradually begin to lift.

Before You Embark on DEMS

If you are currently receiving counselling, the DEMS approach does not have to replace your therapy sessions.

As a practitioner myself, I see the value of in-person sessions, especially the regular follow-up provided by a therapist in your journey towards wellness. That said, this book can be used in accompaniment to your counselling.

The DEMS approach also does not intend to replace any medication prescribed by your doctor. Before you embark on DEMS, do consult your doctor on the suitability of its four components to your current condition or medical treatment.

Please note

This book is not intended to be a substitute for professional diagnosis, treatment or therapy. Be sure to seek the advice of your doctor or mental health provider with any questions you may have regarding your symptoms and condition. If you are working through this book and find that things are getting worse rather than better, do get professional help immediately.

Chapter Summary & Homework

This chapter provided a brief overview of the DEMS approach. A strong and effective dam that can keep flood waters at bay is used as a metaphor for a personal wellness plan that can enhance your mental fortitude and prevent psychological flooding. The DEMS acronym points to the four components of a healthy diet (**D**), participating in engaging activities (**E**), incorporating mindfulness practices (**M**) and having ample sleep (**S**).

Every chapter in this book ends with a set of recommended homework (in the "**Try This**" section) where you get to reflect on key learning and work towards implementing your personal DEMS plan. While the term "homework" may conjure certain memories your time in grade school or university, I would like to encourage you to embrace it in a positive light.

The concept of "homework" in this book is built on the premise that the enhancement of your personal well-being is only possible when knowledge is transferred from your mind to your actions. In the field of psychotherapy and counselling, studies found that clients who do their "homework" between sessions reported significant improvement in their situation compared to those who don't. The DEMS approach that you will soon learn about is only effective to the extent its four components are applied in your daily living. That's why it is my hope that you can attempt the self-reflection questions and tasks recommended in the respective "Try This" sections.

You're in the driver's seat of the change you hope to see.

Remember

Who you are tomorrow begins with what you do today.

- Tim Fargo

Try This!

As you get started on your journey towards a better personal well-being, reflect on the following questions. After reading each question, pause and think deeply about it. Take your time. Notice your thoughts as they come, but refrain from labelling those thoughts as "good" or "bad".

1. Imagine yourself two years from today. Describe what you would be i) feeling, ii) thinking and iii) doing after having achieved an improved mental and emotional well-being.

2.   What are some key reasons for wanting to enhance
     your personal well-being?

3.   Where are you right now with regards to what you
     are i) feeling, ii) thinking and iii) doing?

4. There's a Swedish parable of a little kitten running
    around in circles chasing its own tail. An old cat
    came around and asked what it was doing. The kitten
    replied, "I was told that my tail is my happiness. So,
    I'm trying to catch my happiness." The old cat
    smiled and said, "When I was young, I was told the
    same thing. I spent days and days trying to catch it. I
    became exhausted and in despair. So, I quit and
    moved on with my life… only to discover that my
    tail was there all along, following me."

Is there anything you're chasing after that is tiring
you out?

Tips – Journal your journey

- Writing down your reflections, ideas and plans can be a good way of keeping track of your progress and making them more salient. You may use the space provided in this book, or pen them in a separate journal.

- Off-loading thoughts from your mind onto paper can also provide some forms of clarity and relief.

- Remember to keep your journal and personal DEMS plan somewhere visible and accessible, so that you can review them regularly.

2
D: Diet

On days when Pam's anxiety was more overwhelming, her appetite was also affected. She could go through the day with just a slice of bread and a few glasses of water. Despite reminders from her colleagues and friends to eat, food was just not the most important thing in her mind. The lack of food and water caused her to feel weak and unable to concentrate. In turn, Pam became more susceptible to psychological flooding.

Studies have found that anxiety, depression and stress trigger hormonal and biological changes in your body. These changes can affect your digestive system and make you lose your appetite. You could also be so preoccupied with what's going on in your mind that you might not feel hunger or thirst.

Regardless of your appetite, it is important to remind yourself that food is fuel for your body and nutrition for your brain. A healthy and balanced diet can put you in a better state to manage psychological flooding when it comes.

When you hear the word "diet", you might associate it with eating sparingly or a particular fad diet that is touted to help with weight loss and healthier living. In the field of nutritional science today, there are many fad diets being researched on and promoted (e.g. low carbs, keto, vegan, intermittent fasting, etc.). Information on these diets is widely available in bookstores, libraries and the internet. That said, it is not the purpose of this book to go into these specific diets or recommend any of them. If you have plans to embark on a particular diet, do consult your doctor or dietician to assess if it is suitable for your current health condition.

In the DEMS approach, the term "diet" it is used as a reference to general, habitual nourishment. This chapter focuses on diet in relation to your mental and emotional well-being. Three areas are explored:

- Regular meals

- Mood-boosting foods

- Ample hydration

Let's take a deeper look at each of these aspects.

Regular Meals

Food is one of the most basic needs for humans. It sustained the existence of humans through the ages. The nutrients that food provides is the fuel for us to move and grow. Essential bodily functions, such as breathing, digesting, keeping warm and fighting infections, will start to collapse in the absence of adequate nourishment.

Besides physical growth, food also nourishes us with the mental energy required to develop our minds and manage our emotions. This is all the more important in a world filled with increasing stress and emotional strain.

Keith understood this point well. He noticed he would get more irritable whenever he had to work through lunch or sit in a long meeting without breaks. Initially, he thought it was the work that was contributing to his frustration. As we reviewed his routine, Keith became aware that hunger played a part in affecting his moods. You see, the term "hangry" – a combination of being hungry and angry – isn't just a clever play of words. The popular saying "a hungry man is an angry man" has a physiological explanation behind it.

Studies found that if you haven't eaten for a while, the drop in your blood sugar level interferes with the brain functions related to impulse control, emotional regulation and decision making. When your body detects low blood sugar, it triggers the release of hormones, including cortisol (a stress hormone). While the hormones serve to rebalance your blood sugar, the rise in cortisol levels can also result in irritability, difficulties concentrating and mood swings. Sara Milne Rowe (2018) recounted a particular study that appears to show how some judges' court decisions were affected by their diet. Chances of accused persons getting parole were found to be higher right after meal breaks, and decreased as the time wore on. One deduction was that the food and snacks gave a much-needed boost in their blood sugar levels, making them less testy. In this regard, it doesn't hurt for someone to squeeze their case in after lunch for better chances of parole!

This is not to say that we should overeat, which can lead to negative health consequences. Nutritionists generally recommend going for frequent, smaller meals rather than eating one or two larger ones. What does this look like? Think three balanced meals and one to three light snacks spread throughout the day.

Balanced meals: Calories are basically the measure of energy that food supplies. Depending on your age, weight, height and level of activity, the calories for each main meal could vary between 300 to 600. For a balanced diet, consider limiting your consumption of "empty calories", which are foods that offer minimal nutrition. Cakes, pizza, chips and processed meats are some examples of these foods. Instead, food choices should be well-balanced from the key food groups – vegetables, dairy, grains and proteins.

Light snacks: Having a small nibble between meals can help curb hunger, maintain your blood sugar levels, and enable you to function with a healthier level of mind as you go about your day. Aim for between 100 to 200 calories per snack. Healthy snacks include fresh fruits, whole-wheat bread and nuts. These foods provide more nourishment for your body compared to ice cream, donuts or cookies. That said, being too rigid or restrictive on your diet might be sometimes be counter-productive. Nutritionists and psychologists found that the occasional indulgence on a slice of chocolate cake (or your comfort food) can go a long way in motivating you and helping you stick to a healthy diet plan!

Remember

Vitamin B-12 and other B vitamins, which are present in a well-balanced diet, can aid Serotonin production and mood regulation. Low levels of B vitamins may be linked to depression.

After Keith discovered the importance of not going for too long without food, he made it a point to keep some light snacks in his drawer that he could munch on in between meals. And if he had to work through lunch, he would get a colleague to grab him a sandwich on the way back. Having regular meals, as Keith realised, should not be an endeavour left to chance. If you don't plan for it, you might end up missing your meals.

Here's a list of things that some others have tried. Have a go and see if they work for you too!

- Plan in-advanced where and what to eat.

- Have a hearty breakfast for a good start to the day.

- Avoid going for more than five hours in the day without eating.

- Limit the snacks so your appetite for the main meals is not affected.

- Intentionally cease thinking about your work and enjoy your lunch away from your desk.

- Have a bite before a long meeting, and plan for ample breaks in-between.

- Avoid making important decisions on an empty stomach.

- Arrange to have meals with someone.

Mood-Boosting Foods

Research on the relationship between nutrition and mental health has been emerging in recent years. There are certain foods that have mind-nourishing and mood-boosting properties. They are linked to an increased production of "feel-good chemicals", such as endorphins, serotonin and dopamine, in your body system. As such, they have a direct relation to keeping psychological flooding at bay. Here, we survey two key types of foods that can help you achieve a better brain health.

Omega-3 fatty acids

Omega-3 fatty acids are a family of fatty acids, or polyunsaturated fats, that play an important function in enhancing the fluidity of the cell membrane in your brain. Studies found that regular intake of omega-3 fatty acids lowers the risk of inflammatory diseases and mood disorders. Some have called omega-3 a natural anti-depressant as they improve the circuits of the "feel-good chemicals" in your brain.

While essential to your brain health, your body does not provide these fatty acids on its own – you need to obtain them through your diet! There are three main types of omega-3 fatty acids. **Alpha-linolenic acid (ALA)** is found naturally in plant foods, such as:

- kale,

- spinach,

- soybeans

- chia seeds,

- flaxseeds, and

- walnuts.

Eicosapentaenoic acid (EPA) and **docosahexaenoic acid (DHA)** are mainly found in fatty fish and other seafood, including:

- salmon,

- mackerel,

- herring,

- tuna,

- shrimp, and

- eel.

If your do not have these foods in your diet, you can consider taking an omega-3 supplement, which can be commonly found in health food stores and pharmacies. These include:

- fish oil

- krill oil

- cod liver oil

To achieve an anti-depressant effect, experts recommend (for adults) omega-3 supplements that provide you with 1000mg of EPA and 500mg of DHA per day (Ilardi 2010). As EPA and DHA come from animal products, vegetarians and vegans can consider getting their omega-3 from ALA supplements, such as algal oil and flaxseed oil. However, do bear in mind that your body needs to convert ALA into EPA or DHA before it can be used. And this conversion process is highly inefficient – only a very small percentage of ALA eventually becomes EPA or DHA in your body.

Fermented foods

Apart from omega-3 fatty acids, which are highly recommended, fermented foods have also been touted to contain mood-boosting properties. Up to 90% of your body's serotonin is created in your gut! Emerging research have shown that a healthy gut can contribute towards increased serotonin production and a healthier level of mind. And *probiotics*, which are live microorganisms that enables the growth of healthy bacteria in your gut, is critical for that to happen. Depression symptoms have been found to be lowered after regular consumption of probiotics. Probiotics are formed when foods such as these go through the fermentation process:

- yogurt,

- kimchi,

- pickled vegetables,

- buttermilk,

- kombucha,

- sauerkraut, and

- kefir.

Other fermented foods, such as wine, beer or some types of bread, are not as beneficial as the amount of probiotics is significantly reduced due to filtering and cooking.

Probiotics are also available commercially as a dietary supplement. There are actually many different strains of probiotics. The Lactobacillus and Bifidobacterium strains have been frequently studied in relation to mental health, and are reported to have the most beneficial effects compared to the other strains. If you are going for probiotics supplements, this could be something you want to consider.

Please note

If you are immunocompromised, there is a possibility that you could get an infection – bacteremia or fungemia – from consuming probiotic supplements. Consult your doctor before starting a course of probiotics.

Ample Hydration

Besides having regular, balanced meals and eating foods with mood-boosting properties, it is also essential to ensure you drink enough water for the day. Water is involved in all cellular process in your body. It helps get rid of wastes, regulate your body temperature, lubricate your joints and support metabolism. About 60% of the adult human body and 80% of the brain is comprised of water! Staying hydrated is not just important for your physical well-being, it also helps you to maintain a healthier level of mind.

Enhances efficiency of brain cells: Your brain cells need a certain composition of water and various elements to operate optimally. Ample hydration will help in your cognitive functions, including mental clarity, memory, focus and decision-making. In the absence of adequate hydration, the efficiency of these brain cells is reduced. This can affect your performance at work or ability to interact with others.

Improves moods: Because your brain is made up mostly of water, being even slightly dehydrated can result in headaches, fatigue, confusion and adversely affect your moods. Your mind may not be as agile to notice the onset of psychological flooding and manage rumination. Studies have shown that people who drank more water had a lower risk of anxiety and depression than those who drank less water. Adequate hydration is an important piece of the puzzle for better mental health and emotional regulation.

How much is enough?

You might have come across the advice to drink 6 to 8 glasses of water each day for optimal health. This comes up to around 2.7 to 3.7 liters. There's no one-size-fits-all amount. More specifically, the amount of water you need will vary depending on your weight, level of activity, the climate in which you live in and health condition. Thanks to the internet, you can now find online calculators to ascertain how much water you require based on these variables. Try searching for "water intake calculator" or "hydration calculator". Here's the gist of how these variables corelate with hydration.

Weight: A person weighing 80 kilograms and another weighing 40 kilograms will require different amount of water. Because 60% of our body weight is made of water, the more someone weighs, the more water they need to drink to support bodily functions.

Activity level: If you do activities that make you sweat, you will require more water to cover fluid-loss compared to someone who is more sedentary in the day. And always remember to hydrate yourself before, during and after a workout!

Climate: Your body will produce more sweat in a hot or humid environment. Increase your water intake accordingly to replenish fluid-loss.

Health condition: Certain health conditions may require you to take more or less water. For instance, you need to increase your water intake if you are running a fever, vomiting or having diarrhoea. If you are pregnant or breast-feeding, more water might be needed for optimal hydration. On the other hand, people with certain kidney conditions might be advised by doctors to restrict their water intake.

One way to know if you are adequately hydrated is to check the colour of your urine. It should be light yellow (pale straw) in colour. Urine that is darker in colour is an indication of dehydration, while clear or colourless urine can mean that you are drinking more than you should – a sign that you can cut back. If unsure, your doctor or dietitian can help you determine the amount of water that's sufficient for you.

Do note your daily hydration does not come solely from the beverages you drink. On average, around 20% of daily fluid intake comes from food and the rest from drinks. Many fruits and vegetables are water-rich. For example, watermelons, strawberries, cucumbers and lettuces have a water content of more than 90%! Factor these into your daily diet as well.

Here're some tips to optimise your water intake:

- Don't wait till you are thirsty before you drink up. Thirst is often a sign that you could already be dehydrated, and sometimes accompanied by fatigue and headaches. Instead, drink small amounts of water regularly (e.g. hourly) to ensure ample hydration.

- For better health, go easy on sugar-sweetened drinks which can pile on more calories than required. Consider "plain" water, which can come in the forms of distilled water, filtered water and boiled water, etc.

- Make it a habit to carry a botte of water with you wherever you go.

- Set an alarm on your mobile device to remind you to drink up every hour or so.

- If you want to add flavour, you can try infusing your water with fruits such as lemon, lime or strawberries. Infuser water bottles, which have an inner basket or mesh to contain the fruits, are widely available nowadays.

Please note

Drinking plenty of water each day is one of the simplest forms of self-care there is.

- Claire Chamberlain

Chapter Summary & Homework

In this chapter, you have learnt the importance of how your diet can help enhance your mental and emotional well-being:

- Having regular and balanced meals can help maintain your blood sugar at a level where you are able to better manage your thoughts and emotions.

- Mood-boosting foods such as omega-3 fatty acids can support the production of the "feel-good" chemicals in your brain.

- Ample hydration prevents fatigue, confusion and poor concentration, and enhances the efficiency of your brain cells.

The body energy and mental energy that a nourishing diet brings form the foundation for you to pursue the other components of DEMS. With a healthier level of mind, you will be able to better engage your daily activities, interact with others and care for yourself. Conversely, having low levels of body and mental energy could make you more vulnerable to depression, anxiety and stress.

Try This!

To help you get the Diet (D) component of DEMS in order, try out the following activities this week:

1. What are some of your favourite foods and beverages?

2. How would you describe your current relationship with food?

3. How does your moods affect your diet, and vice versa?

4. On a piece of paper or notebook, create a meal plan
    for the next 3 days that takes into consideration i)
    regular, balanced meals, ii) foods with mood-
    boosting properties, and iii) adequate hydration. If
    your current diet already consists of these things,
    plan how you could improve on it.

5. Carry out your meal plan (see item 4), then spend
    some time reflecting on the following questions. It
    doesn't matter if you were not able to stick to all that
    you have planned. Remember, be kind and gentle
    with yourself as you reflect.

6. How is this meal plan different from your usual diet?

7. Which component of your meal plan was easiest to achieve? Why?

8. Which component of your meal plan was most
    challenging to stick to? Why?

9. Go through the lists of strategies and tips in this
    chapter. Select those which you want to implement
    as part of your personal DEMS plan (in chapter 6).

3
E: Engaging Activities

Have you ever experienced your thoughts spiralling out of control? This could come in the form of overthinking a decision, excessive worrying or stressing over a particular situation. Without a strategy to keep it in check and reign in the train of thoughts, psychological flooding can take place. And it often happens without you being consciously aware of it.

Why is that so?

Many a times, engaging in those thoughts, also known as rumination, seems like a natural thing to do. Your brain may be driven by some of these underlying beliefs:

- "I have a decision to make. Of course, I need to give it some thought."

- "This issue is important to me. So, it's natural I am worried about it."

- "It is part and parcel of problem-solving."

- "Thinking about the worst-case scenario will help me be more prepared… and perhaps reduce the hurt when it eventually happens."

There are also external factors that create opportunities for rumination, such as:

- Unstructured free time.

- Mentally draining activities.

- Lack of social support.

While a healthy amount of contemplation is essential, ruminating can affect your daily functioning, especially when you become a prisoner of your thoughts. Rumination can become a loop – the more you submerse in it, the harder it is to snap out of it.

Engaging activities can help you manage those straying thoughts.

What are Engaging Activities

Engaging activities – the "E" component of DEMS – are activities that keep your mind *occupied, energized* or both! Let me briefly unpack what these two terms mean:

An occupied mind: When performing a task, your mind is occupied by the present moment experiences instead of straying with rumination. This concept is covered in greater detail in Chapter 5 when I talk about *mindfulness*[1]. For now, here're some examples of being mentally occupied by the task at hand.

- While filing papers at work, you think about the order of filing and focus on sorting out the papers in the correct order.

- While jogging around the park, you concentrate on your breathing and the movement of your legs and arms.

- While watching a movie, you engross yourself in the plot and admire the cinematography.

Think of your mind as a cup. When the cup is full, there is no room to add more water into it. Similarly, the

---

[1] In Chapter 4 (Mindfulness), specific principles and techniques of mindfulness will be touched on. The concept of mindfulness partially underpins the engaging activities you'll learn about in this chapter. Apart from mindfulness in action, engaging activities also achieve distinct physiological, mental and emotional benefits. Hence, it is given its own spot in the DEMS approach.

more mentally engaged you are in an activity, the lesser room you have in your mind for rumination.

An energised mind: While mundane tasks can occupy your mind, they may or may not energise it. Activities that supply mental energy to our minds are those that:

- Trigger the release of feel-good brain chemicals such as serotonin.

- Create interest, curiosity and pleasure.

- Boost our moods.

You'll learn about some of these activities in a while.

Now, you may be wondering – isn't mentally engaging activities a form of distraction or avoidance from our thoughts? When the activities are over, won't reality hit and the thoughts come back?

Well, yes and no.

As you'll pick up in the next chapter, mindfulness is not about avoiding certain thoughts or emotions – avoidance can result in other challenges and those suppressed feelings might leak out in other unhelpful ways. Rather, you can acknowledge and accept the presence of these thoughts in your mind (*Ok, I'm having these thoughts right now*), but refrain from analysing it for the time being. In shifting your awareness from rumination to the task at hand, you sidestep what could potentially be a draining and destructive downward spiral.

The thing is this – the more your mind is accustomed to switching from ruminating to engaging in an activity, the more adept you will be in keeping your thoughts from drifting when you are not doing any tasks. Like muscle memory, this takes practice.

Tip – Limit the Ruminate

Instead of giving in to rumination whenever it comes, intentionally schedule a slot (of no more than ten minutes) each day to worry and stress over a particular issue. When the time is up, move away from that state of rumination to focus on your next task.

There are many types of engaging activities you can participate in. In the following sections, I will talk about three categories of activities and highlight some benefits that each can have on your mental and emotional well-being:

- Work

- Exercise

- Leisure

Work

Have you ever had the experience of being so engrossed in your work that the personal problem you were ruminating about earlier on disappeared from your mind? This shows two things. First, doing work can engage your mind while putting your skills and talents to good use. Second, the "problem" you were thinking about was, to an extent, a product of your thoughts – ruminating about it could have made it appear bigger and more real than it actually was.

Depending on the nature of your job, work can take up anywhere from 10 to more than 50 hours of our week. That's a significant amount of time! Studies have found that work satisfaction can affect our mental health. Whether you are a freelancer, office worker or a stay-at-home parent, doing work which you enjoy can increase your satisfaction and personal well-being. By contrast, people who are less happy in their jobs report lower mental health scores and are more susceptible to depression, anxiety and stress.

Ideally, we want to experience fulfilment from our work. In reality, however, work tops the list of stress triggers in adults. Around the world, work-related stresses account for high burn-out rates. Navigating the stresses related to work can reap tremendous benefits. Regardless of whether you see your job as a calling, a source of income or an advancement of career, you can manage how you go about your work in order to be more mentally engaged and curb rumination.

Get organised: A big project or a looming deadline can be stress-inducing. Plan and prioritise the work that needs to be done. Breaking down a task into bite sized portions makes work more manageable and reduces stress levels.

Reduce multi-tasking: Doing too much at once not only affects productivity, but can create stress and anxiety. As such, work becomes less engaging and more mentally draining. After breaking down the work into smaller portions, focus on one task at a time. Allow yourself to enjoy the satisfaction of completing each task, however simple it might be.

Get started: Sometimes, we get overwhelmed by the thoughts about what needs to be done and how to tackle the tasks. Spending too much time overthinking about work can lead to "analysis paralysis", which is a form of psychological flooding. When you sense that you are starting to overthink about the tasks, try doing something to get things started. The journey of a thousand miles begins with a single step.

Tip

Taking breaks of ten to fifteen minutes away from your work can leave you feeling refreshed and better able to engage the task at hand.

Exercise

When it comes to exercising, I'll admit I'm not an expert. I do not participate in team sports. And I do not hit the gym either. My exercise fix comprises of a 30-minute jog to the beach and back, two to three times a week. It usually takes longer if I slow to a walk. But this much I can tell you – exercise provides energy not just for the body, but also has profound neurological and psychological benefits for your brain.

Exercise is medicine!

Here are some key benefits of exercising in relation to our mental and emotional well-being.

Occupies the mind: Exercises that require fixed repetitive movement, such as walking, swimming, jogging or cycling, can keep our minds mentally engaged on those motions. This means lesser chance of rumination taking place while you are concentrating on your swim strokes or jogging strides.

Regulates moods: Any forms of physical work out can trigger the release of feel-good brain chemicals such as endorphins, dopamine and serotonin. These brain chemicals serve to lift our moods and enhance mental agility. This is especially so with aerobic exercises – cardiovascular activities which increases your breathing and heart rate. Aerobic exercises are found to have antidepressant effects when performed for about 30-40 minutes three times a week.

Improves appetite and sleep: Apart from lifting moods, serotonin also helps to improve your appetite and sleep cycles, which can be adversely affected when you are going through mentally and emotionally challenging times. Thus, exercise can contribute towards building the D (diet) and S (sleep) components of DEMS. And vice versa!

Reduces stress: Regular exercise balances the level of stress hormones, such as adrenalin, in our body system. This enables you to cope better under stressful situations instead of being psychologically flooded.

Remember

Physical movement is part of who we are. As humans, we are meant to move… Being in better physical shape might help us manage a tricky conversation, for example, or focus for longer on a document, or have more patience.

- Sara Milne Rowe

I'm guessing here that most people probably know that exercise is good for them. But many find it a challenge to do it regularly enough for them to experience the benefits of it. Let's take a look at two common barriers to regular exercise and possible strategies to overcome them.

Barrier 1: The Time Factor

In today's busy world, many of my clients find it a challenge to fit exercise into their schedule. Even after paying thousands of dollars for a yearly gym membership, they visit the gym only once or twice a month due to the demands of work and family life. The lack of exercise, in turn, affects their ability to manage the stresses bought about by those demands.

Solution: While planning and prioritising your work tasks and family commitments, make it a point to slot in periods of exercise and physical activities into your weekly schedule. There will always be things on your plate. But I like how one of my clients put it – *something's gotta give!* Make exercise a priority, even if you struggle to find your momentum initially.

Use the personal DEMS plan template at the end of Chapter 6 to schedule time for exercise. Remember, going to the gym is not the only way to be active. Think about how you can incorporate general movement throughout the day. Here's what some people tried and found helpful:

- "My work is quite sedentary. So, I set a timer on my watch that will sound every hour in the day. I then proceed to do some stretches or take a walk around the office each time."

- "Instead of alighting at my bus stop when I come home from work, I now get off two stops before and take a stroll home."

- "I had a discussion with my spouse around household chores and child-care arrangements, and carved out Monday and Thursday evenings to attend yoga sessions."

- "I now wake up an hour earlier – before my wife and children – in order to exercise. I was initially hesitant as I thought it might sap my energy and make me feel tired while at work. Instead, I was able to focus a lot better."

- "I live in a high-rise apartment, and I have taken to climbing the stairs instead of using the elevator."

Barrier 2: The Motivation Factor

Having low levels of energy is one of the symptoms of depression and anxiety. You may feel weak, lethargic and unmotivated to do anything. In such a state, getting a work out may require a lot of effort and willpower. In the absence of any forms of work out, the lack of body and mental energy that exercise provides can create a vicious cycle – you feel weaker and, in turn, more unmotivated to get anything done.

Solution: Set smaller goals for the initial period. Baby steps, if you like. It could be a 5-minute walk around your neighbourhood. Or simple stretches on the mat in your bedroom. Once you get started, the increased energy will, in turn, enhance your moods and motivation. Creating some form of external accountability can also improve your chances of achieving your exercise goals. This includes:

- Sharing your exercise schedule with a trusted friend and enlist his or her support in keeping you accountable.

- Making arrangements to exercise with your friends or partner.

- Using fitness apps on your device that track your progress.

While plans can be made, there will be times when you do not carry it through. Especially when the low moods seem very overwhelming. When that happens, don't beat yourself up for failing to get moving. Instead, gently notice the thoughts and emotions that surface during those moments. For some, it might be guilt or disappointment. For others, it might be a sense of lethargy or laziness. Acknowledge those feelings without dwelling too much on it. Then, move on to schedule a future session to exercise.

Remember

It always seems impossible until it's done.

- Nelson Mandela

Leisure

There is more to life than just attending to work, personal or family responsibilities. We need downtime or "me time", as some may call it, to engage in leisure and recharge ourselves. Leisure activities bring you enjoyment and pleasure. Even small and simple things can add up to help you feel better. Leisure could take the form of:

A hobby – Picking up a healthy hobby helps your mind to be meaningfully occupied and maintain a sense of curiosity. While engaging in your hobby, give it your full attention. Whether it's making music, home improvement, brewing coffee or solving Sudoku, studies have found that people with hobbies are less likely to buckle under depression, anxiety and stress.

An outing – Activities that get you out and about can improve your mental and emotional well-being. Outings can comprise of activities done indoors, such as a visit to museum or a walk in the mall, or outdoors, like the beach or park. Spending time in nature has been found to promote cognitive functions and overall well-being. Doing something outdoors where you get exposure to sunlight has the added benefit of increased serotonin levels in your brain. While too much of sunlight can be harmful to the skin, around 30-minutes of sunlight exposure each day can be mood-boosting. Just don't forget the sunscreen!

Inject Leisure, Break the Stress Cycle

Many of us tend to stop doing leisure activities when we are feeling low or stressed. It could be a challenging situation in your career or a turn of events in your personal life. While it may seem counter-intuitive to have fun when you are pressurised by the demands of life, removing leisure can perpetuate a stress cycle. Take for instance this work-related stress cycle:

1.   You performed below expectations at work.

2.   You feel stressed.

3.   You stop doing things you enjoy (leisure activities).

4.   Your self-concept and moods are affected because of the absence of enjoyment.

5.   Your performance dips.

6.   You feel more stressed (cycle repeats).

Solution: The next time you find yourself in a challenging situation, you can potentially break the stress cycle by injecting leisure activities, however little, into your routine. The pleasure, relaxation and fun that accompanies leisure activities can improve your self-concept and moods, which contribute towards enhanced creativity and productivity.

Of course, we're not talking about engaging in so much leisure that it eats into our working hours or family time. Use the personal DEMS plan template at the end of Chapter 6 to inject some leisure into your schedule.

Nourishing, Draining or Both?

Activities that you do throughout the day – work, exercise, leisure and other daily routines – can be classified as nourishing or draining. Nourishing activities energise your mind and lift your moods, while draining activities sap your mental energy away. In fact, some activities can be both nourishing and draining at the same time! For example, doing household chores is nourishing for me as it feels good living in a clean and tidy home. But it also draining as I can be tired out by the cleaning.

We are usually more mentally engaged if an activity is nourishing, and less engaged if it is draining. It is recommended you do a stocktake of your daily routine to have a sense of how each activity is impacting your mental energy and personal well-being.

We will now take a look at how Keith applied this to his regular weekday routine.

Case Study – Keith

Let's turn our attention back to Keith, who was trying to manage work-related stress and achieve better work-life balance. During one of our coaching sessions, Keith listed down his workday routine and labelled those activities as nourishing (N), draining (D) or both (ND).

- Wash up – N
- Dress up – N
- Have breakfast – N
- Drive to work – D
- Type emails and reports – D
- Have lunch – N
- Attend meetings – D
- Drive home from work – D
- Bathe – N
- Have dinner – N
- Spend time with family – N
- Listen to music – N

To enhance your personal well-being, there are a few things you can do in your daily routine:

1. Increase the number of nourishing activities

2. Reduce the number of draining activities (provided it is within your control).

3. For draining activities that cannot be avoided, you can reduce the impact the draining activity has on your mental energy by pairing it with a nourishing one.

Let's go back to Keith to see how this works.

Case Study – Keith (continue)

Having done a stocktake of his daily routine, Keith found driving to work to be draining due to the heavy traffic. Work-related tasks such as typing emails and reports also became increasingly draining as the increased workload and demanding expectations snuff out some of the passion he once had.

Wishing to be more mentally engaged while at work, Keith strategised to pair some of the draining activities with nourishing ones:

- Listen to his favourite tunes (N) while driving (D) and at work (D).

- Take regular short breaks away from his desk (N) while typing reports and emails (D) and after a long meeting (D).

- Have a 5-minute phone conversation with his wife and children (N) in the middle of the work day.

These strategies worked for Keith, who found his time at work to be more "bearable". Gradually, his perception about work became more positive, along with a reduced sense of dread.

Chapter Summary & Homework

In this chapter, you have learnt how certain activities are engaging and nourishing to the mind. Being mentally engaged by doing work, exercise and leisure activities boosts your personal well-being in several ways:

- Focusing on the task in front of you, however mundane it might be, leaves lesser room in your mind for other worries or concerns.

- Regular exercise and being out in the sun improve moods through triggering the release of feel-good chemicals in the brain.

- Engaging in leisure activities, such as a hobby or an outing, injects pleasure into your daily routine and breaks the cycle of stress.

- Pairing draining activities with nourishing ones can make them more mentally engaging.

While it can be challenging to focus on these activities when you are feeling down or stressed, taking baby steps and celebrating every small accomplishment can go a long way in building your DEMS.

Try This!

1. What about your work do you find satisfying? What about it is stress-inducing?

2. How has anxiety, depression or stress interfered with your performance at work?

3. What exercise/s will you commit to do this week?
    When and where will you be doing it?

4. What are your barriers to regular exercise? What are
    some strategies you can put in place to overcome
    these barriers?

5. Doing things which make you feel good should be on your weekly routine! What leisure activities trigger your interest? (Note: These could be activities you are currently doing or those you have yet to try.)

6. How does your moods affect your level of exercise and leisure, and vice versa?

7. On a piece of paper, list down your daily routine in chronological order – things you do from the moment you wake up to your bedtime. Label each activity "N" (nourishing), "D" (draining) or "ND" (both nourishing and draining). Review your list, and think about how you can:

- Increase the "N" activities.

- Reduce the "D" activities.

- If you can't reduce the "D" activities, how can you modify them or pair them up with "N" activities to make them more engaging?

8. Go through the tips and suggestions in this chapter. Select those which you will implement in your personal DEMS plan (in chapter 6).

4
M: Mindfulness

Grant me the serenity to accept the things I cannot change, Courage to change the things I can, And wisdom to know the difference.

Serenity Prayer

In the previous chapters, we learnt that rumination can cause our thoughts to spiral out of control. Depending on whether you are experiencing depression, anxiety or stress, mental rumination can assume various forms.

Firstly, our minds might dwell on past events – we beat ourselves up for the things that went wrong, and constantly regret over what could have been.

Secondly, our minds might anticipate problems that might happen in the future – we worry about the worst-case scenarios and contemplate all the possible solutions in advance.

You might think that analysing it over and over again can help you solve the problem, or at least bring you closer to a solution. In reality, however, it might be akin to flooring the accelerator when your car is stuck in the mud – it brings you nowhere. And you might be sucked deeper in.

The effective management of rumination can prevent psychological flooding from running its course. This is where mindfulness comes in.

What is Mindfulness

Instead of dwelling on the past or the future, mindfulness enables us to focus our awareness on the *here and now*. We intentionally pay attention to the present moment in a non-judgemental manner. Let me briefly unpack some of the key words in the previous sentence.

Intentionally – Mindfulness requires a deliberate effort on our part. Through repeated practice, the way our brains respond to events and triggers can be altered and mindfulness becomes a more natural process.

Pay attention – This is more of a *noticing* posture rather than going into an analysing or problem-solving mode. We simply acknowledge what we are experiencing within and around us in the present moment.

Present moment – The present moment comprises of our physical sensations, emotions and thoughts. For example, if you are seated on the couch, you can focus your awareness on:

- the sensation of your back leaning against the cushion.

- the feeling of your feet resting against the floor.

- the coolness of the air on your skin.

- the sounds from the surrounding entering your ears.

One key aspect of mindfulness is bringing awareness to your breath, which is present with you wherever you are. While breathing is usually an unconscious behaviour, we can become more mindful of it by paying attention to:

- the sensation of the air entering and leaving your nostrils.

- the rising and falling of your abdomen with your in-breath and out-breath.

- the sounds you make when breathing.

Non-judgemental – When thoughts enter our minds, we practice non-judgement by temporarily setting aside the urge to do something about those thoughts. We accept the presence of these thoughts in our minds for what they are – thoughts, not facts. By not judging those thoughts as "good" or "bad", the chances of reacting to our thoughts are reduced. We do not yearn after the "good" thoughts, or attempt to fix or hide from the "bad" ones. Being non-judgemental also means:

- Being gentle and kind to yourself, rather than beating yourself up.

- Accepting yourself as who you are, instead of trying to be someone else.

Being Aware We Have a Thought

When you are feeling down, negative thoughts and beliefs can be awakened. You might find yourself being caught up in old habits of the mind – certain trains of thought that you are prone to ruminate on. You could even, whether consciously or subconsciously, believe those thoughts to be true because of how they fit with how you feel. Your low moods and rumination then influence each other, activating a downward spiral. Consider the following cycle:

- Your mood dips.

- Negative thoughts surface.

- Your mood dips even more.

- More negative thoughts surface (cycle repeats).

Through mindfulness, you notice the initial dips in your moods and pull yourself out before getting enveloped in full blown negativity.

Now, the goal of mindfulness is not to empty the mind. We cannot stop thoughts and feelings from arising – our brains are naturally wired to have thoughts. Our thoughts are also part of our *here and now* experience. Avoiding thoughts or being afraid of them can increase anxiety instead.

That said, it's important to note that you are not your thoughts. And not all thoughts are helpful. Just because a thought comes up in your mind doesn't mean it's true – thoughts are thoughts, not facts. Epistemologically speaking, the past is made of memories (often influenced by your perceptions of events), and the future has yet to arrive (so no one knows for sure what would happen).

There's also a possibility that the thought you have could actually be what is known as a "cognitive distortion" – a misleading and often inaccurate way of thinking about yourself, others and the world. As you go through the following list of some common cognitive distortions, try and see if you can identify which are the ones your mind is more susceptible to.

- **All-or-nothing thinking**: You view situations, people or yourself in absolute or extreme categories. They're either good or bad, positive or negative. This can be unhelpful as reality often exists between the two extremes.

- **Overgeneralization**: You take a conclusion about one event and apply that for other situations in life. For example, if you went through a failed relationship, you might think that any future relationships will suffer the same fate.

- **Mental filtering**: You have a tendency to focus on the negatives and ignore the positives.

- **Mind reading**: You assume what other people are thinking without any concrete evidence. This often involves assuming that they are reactively negatively towards you.

- **Catastrophising**: You assume the worst about a situation, believing that things will turn out badly. Things could be blown way out of proportion.

- **Personalisation**: You take things personally when they are not connected to you or caused by you.

- **Labelling**: You use a negative label or descriptor on yourself or others. For example, instead of saying, "I made a mistake," you tell yourself, "I'm a failure."

- **Blame**: You blame yourself for something you were not entirely responsible for. Blame can also be attributed to other people or events.

Many of these cognitive distortions are associated with heightened depression, anxiety or stress. In this regard, treating all your thoughts as reality might do you a disservice.

Coming back to Pam's experience – when she felt a little short of breath while walking home, the thought that she might be having a heart attack flooded her mind. As that thought appeared real to her, Pam began feeling nervous. Because of her nervousness, her heart started beating faster and her breathing became more rapid. These physiological sensations, in turn, led her to believe more strongly that something was wrong with her heart.

Keith, who was worried about his job security, was also in such a situation with his thoughts. Whenever his boss scheduled a meeting with him or called him into her office, Keith would think that he was going to be retrenched or dismissed. The more he thought about that scenario, the more intense his fears grew. He began interpreting things as signs that he was going to be made redundant – colleagues talking behind his back, a mistake he made in a recent report, another colleague being given an important assignment instead of him, etc. Even though those events might not have meant anything much, Keith's perceptions became his version of reality, escalating his stress and anxiety levels.

The thoughts you have can have immense influence on your physical and emotional states. You feel the way you think! Through practising the mindfulness techniques that you will learn about in this chapter, Pam and Keith were able to relate to their thoughts differently, and prevent the down spiral which their ruminations used to take them.

One of the ways which mindfulness can change how you relate to you thoughts is by seeing your thoughts through an *observer's mind.*

Observer's mind – When a thought or feeling comes about, try viewing it like how an observer would. That is, from a third-party perspective. For example, instead of thinking "I am not able to do this", you tell yourself "I see I have a thought that I am not able to do this". One technique to carry this out is to view your thoughts as if you are watching a movie on the screen. By practising this distanced observing, you start to relate to your thoughts as temporary mental events that are separate from yourself and not necessarily an accurate reflection of reality.

How to Bring Awareness to the Present?

Instead of suppressing the thoughts that surface, you simply notice and acknowledge them non-judgmentally from an observer's perspective ("Okay, I notice I'm having this thought", "So, this is what I am feeling right now.").

What you could suppress, though, is the urge to judge, analyse or fix every thought that come along. To facilitate that, you direct your attention back to your breath or use any of your five senses – touch, sound, sight, smell and taste – to connect you to the present moment (see section on Mindfulness Practices). This is also known as *grounding*.

If the thought re-surfaces, you simply acknowledge its presence ("Oh, that thought is here again.", "Interesting… I can sense this emotion in me again.") and gently bring your attention back to the original object of your awareness once again.

This process can be summed up using the acronym **NAS** – *Notice, Acknowledge, Shift*:

- Notice when thoughts arise.

- Acknowledge them non-judgementally using an observer's mind.

- Shift your attention back to your object of awareness.

When your mind wanders off again, as all minds do, just repeat the NAS process and keep bringing your awareness back to the point of focus.

Developing the skill of mindfulness is like training your muscles – the more practice you have in bringing your awareness back after it wanders, the more adept you will be. Each time you are able to notice your mind wandering, you are building the muscle of *mindful awareness*. Thus, you do not have to feel frustrated or upset at your wandering thoughts, even if it happens over and over again. See it as a chance for practice!

Practising mindfulness doesn't mean the thoughts that popped up or the issues that are happening are swept under the carpet. After doing the mindfulness practices, many people benefit from having better emotional control and clarity of mind. When they revisit the thoughts and issues at a later time, they are in a better state of mind to respond appropriately rather than react in the heat of the moment.

Benefits of Mindfulness

Increasing number of studies in the past decade have shed light into how mindfulness can promote mental and emotional well-being. Some benefits of regular mindfulness practice include:

- Increase in self-compassion and positive affect.

- Reduction in levels of depression, anxiety, stress, worry and anger.

- Improved quality of sleep.

- Improved emotional control.

- Better pain management.

These benefits are accompanied by actual physical changes to our brains. An increase in thickness was documented in the pre-frontal cortex – the part of the brain responsible for concentration and decision-making. The amygdala, which is associated with fear and emotion, was also found to have reduced in size.

All in all, this means we can become more thoughtful in our responses rather than being hijacked by our emotions. Good news for the prevention of psychological flooding!

Mindfulness Practices

The key to making mindfulness a part of your lifestyle is to embed it into the everyday. There are many simple, effective mindfulness exercises to try out. I've shared about how to sit and breathe mindfully in the earlier section on "What is Mindfulness". A few other mindfulness practices are suggested here. They can be implemented in various contexts and do not take up more than 10 minutes each time.

If you are new to mindfulness, these practices might take a bit of getting used to. They are certainly not the usual way we go about doing things. Thoughts such as "Why am I doing this?" or "Does this really work?" might pop up in your brain, as it did in mine when I first tried them out. Simply notice and acknowledge those thoughts. They need not stop you from getting a taste of mindfulness.

So, have a go and see which appeals to you. Then plan how you can customise one or more of them to fit into your routine, even if it is just for a few minutes each day.

Mindful Listening

We might not realise it, but sounds are entering our ears every moment we are awake. In mindful listening, we pause whatever we are doing, and channel some awareness to our sense of hearing. For the next 5 minutes, let sound become the object of your awareness.

- Sit comfortably in a conducive spot where you won't be interrupted.

- Begin by bringing awareness to your breathing. Allow yourself to breathe naturally, and observe your breath as it enters and leaves your body.

- Now, close your eyes and allow the surrounding sounds to flow into your ears.

- Focus on the quality of each sound. Is it loud or soft? Is it near or far? Is it coming or going? Is it low pitched or high pitched? Does it repeat?

- If you notice any thoughts or feelings arise, simply acknowledge them non-judgementally. Then, gently shift your awareness back to the sounds.

- When the time is up, slowly open your eyes and carry on with your daily routine.

Mindful Eating

Eating is such an integral part of our lives. For this exercise, you will be applying your five senses as you eat. A raisin is used here as an example. But the steps can be replicated with any meals you are having. If you usually rush through your meals, now's the time to slow it down a notch or two.

- First, hold the raisin in your hand.

- **Sight**: Take a minute to look at it with curiosity, as if you are seeing it for the first time. Observe the shape, the colours, the patterns, etc.

- **Touch**: Feel the texture of the raisin with your fingers and notice its weight. Observe how its shape changes when you squeeze it.

- **Smell**: Bring it close to your nose and smell it. Is there any particular aroma?

- **Hearing**: Hold it near your ears and give it a tap or a scratch. Listen out for the sounds it produces.

- Now, slowly place the raisin in your mouth.

- **Taste**: Pay attention to its texture and taste as you move it around the different parts of your mouth. What do you also notice about your saliva?

- As you slowly chew and swallow the raisin, does it leave a residual taste in your mouth or your throat?

- If a thought or feeling surfaces any time during this exercise, give it some space and look at it using an observer's mind. After that, invite your awareness back to your physical sensations without needing to fix that thought or emotion.

- Bon appétit!

Mindful Walking

For some of us, taking a walk is an opportunity to think about stuff and, perhaps, do some problem-solving. All's good until our brains go into an overdrive mode. In mindful walking, we consciously bring our awareness to the act of walking itself, one step at a time.

- Find a conducive and safe stretch of passageway for walking. It should allow for you to take around ten steps. If you're indoors, consider going bare footed.

- As you slowly lift up your left leg to walk, notice the sensation of your weight being shifted to your right leg.

- As your left heel slowly lands on the ground, pay close attention to your stride – the roll of your left foot from the heel to the toes.

- Notice when your right heel begins to lift off the ground.

- Take note of how your weight is being distributed from your right leg to your left.

- Repeat the same motion with your right foot and notice the sensations.

- If you feel unsteady or wobble, acknowledge that without judgement.

- If you notice your mind wandering off at any point, simply acknowledge that before returning to what you are focusing on.

If you are taking a stroll outdoors, you can try focusing on an object of awareness (e.g. your stride) for a few minutes before shifting your attention to another focal point using other senses. And you might find that there's aplenty to feast your senses upon! Here are some suggestions:

- As you walk, detect what each of your senses pick up, one bit at a time.

- **Sight**: Look at an object, e.g. the leaves on the tree, the sky, a building, a creature, etc. Notice its every detail – the size, shape, colours and patterns.

- **Hearing**: Concentrate on the sounds flowing into your ears, e.g. rustling of leaves, birds chirping, vehicles moving, footsteps, your breathing, etc.

- **Smell**: Notice the smells picked up by your nose.

- **Touch**: Channel your awareness to your physical sensations, e.g. the rising and falling of your chest and abdomen as you breathe, the trickling of sweat down your forehead, the ambient temperature on your skin, etc.

Tips for Mindful Walking

- Slowing down your pace a little can help you notice your surrounding better.

- Concentrate on one object of awareness at a time.

- Extend a non-judgemental attitude to what your senses pick up.

- The steps in this mindfulness practice can also be applied in other exercises such as jogging or cycling.

- Safety first! Watch out for traffic and hazards on the road.

Being Mindful In Other Daily Activities

By now, you might start to get the gist of mindfulness – bringing your awareness to one focal point and gently cradling it with your attention without judgement. The same mindful posture laid out in the previous exercises can also be applied in other daily activities. For example:

- **Brushing teeth**: Notice the sensations of the bristles on your gums, or how your hand grips the toothbrush.

- **Showering**: Notice the smell of the soap, the temperature of the water, and the feeling of the water on your skin. Observe the bubbles on the foam.

- **Getting dressed**: Notice the sensation of your clothing in contact with your skin.

- **Making coffee**: Pay attention to the aroma. Observe how the steam rises up and disappears into the air. Notice how the coffee swirls as you stir.

- **Mopping the floor**: Take note of how the mop glides across the surface of the floor. Notice the amount of pressure you use to hold the handle.

- **Taking the bus (or train)**: Observe the design and colours of the interior of the bus, or the scenery outside. Listen out for the sounds. Attend mindfully to your breathing.

The Body Scan

In this mindfulness practice, you will systematically move your awareness through your body, starting from your toes to your head. Focus on one area of your body at a time. Spend around a minute attending to each area mindfully, paying close attention to any physical sensations you can pick up.

- Before you begin, give yourself permission to spend the next ten minutes or so to go through this mindfulness exercise – any other tasks or issues can wait.

- Sit comfortably in a quiet and conducive spot, with both feet placed gently on the ground (you may also lie down, if you wish).

- Close your eyes, or keep them half-open (soft focus).

- Pay attention to your in-breath and out-breath for a few moments.

- **Toes**: First, guide your attention to the toes on your feet. See if you can sense each individual toe, and even the spaces between the toes. Refrain from seeing the image of your toes in your mind – simply rely on your bodily sensations.

- **Feet**: Next, move your attention to the soles, heels, ankles and upper part of your feet. Notice any sensations in the muscles, skin or bones in those areas. Chances are your mind might get distracted with a thought or sound. That's fine. It's what the mind does. Just acknowledge that and patiently bring your attention back to your feet.

- **Legs**: From your feet, slowly guide your awareness upwards to your calf, shin, knees and thighs. See if you can notice any pressure from the chair, or sensations from your clothing. Or you might notice that you are not noticing anything. That's a form of noticing too!

- **Torso (lower)**: Now, let go mentally of your legs as best as you can, and shift your attention to your lower torso. Focus on one region at a time, starting with your tailbone and slowly moving your awareness upwards to your hips, lower back and lower abdomen. Notice if there are any sensations in your intestines and stomach.

- **Torso (upper)**: Bring your awareness now to your chest. Notice your heart beating. Feel the air flowing in and out of your lungs. Then shift your attention to your upper back and shoulder blades.

- **Hands**: Letting go mentally of your torso, focus your attention now on both your hands. Start by noticing what your fingers feel like. Then move your attention to your palms and the back of your hands.

- **Arms**: Slowly move your awareness upwards to your wrists, forearms, elbows, upper arms and shoulders. If your mind wanders, gently invite your awareness back to your arms.

- **Neck**: Shift your attention now to your neck. Notice any sensations around your neck and inside your throat. Feel the sensation of air moving in and out of your throat as you breathe.

- **Head**: Continue by shifting your awareness up to your head, starting with your chin, mouth, cheeks, nose, ears, eyes and eye brows. Finally, pay close attention to your forehead and the crown of your head. See if you can notice the sensations of hair and muscles on your scalp.

- Mentally let go of the sensations on your head. Rest in this moment for a while – coming back to your breath – before bringing your awareness back to the room. Slowly allow your eyes to open and stretch if you need to.

Please note

This is not meant to be a relaxation exercise, although feeling relaxed can be a pleasant by-product. The aim of the Body Scan is to shift your awareness to different parts of your body, and noticing the *here and now* without judgement.

If you notice any discomfort in certain areas of your body (e.g. an itch, a sore muscle, etc), try as best as you can to recognise it without trying to fix it on the spot. With regular practice, your ability to acknowledge yet shift your attention away from the discomfort can be transferred to other life situations:

- Some problems in life might not go away. Instead of reacting to it, you can choose how to respond appropriately or work around it.

- If you avoid painful emotions and thoughts, your brain might start to perceive them as a threat. Acknowledging its presence without judgement can make them appear less menacing to your brain.

The 3-Minute Breathing Space

As the name suggests, this mindfulness practice is 3-minute time-out where you can connect with your breath and body. Each minute has a specific focus. If you like, you may set a gentle alarm to signal the end of every minute.

Some people do this short practice in the middle of the work-day as they found it to be a recharging experience. Others slot this in before a meeting or presentation to help them become more collected. I do the 3-minute breathing space before bedtime to wrap up the day.

- Find somewhere private where you won't be disturbed.

- You may do this sitting, standing or lying down. You can also choose to keep your eyes closed, half-closed or open.

- **1st minute – Checking-in**: Mentally notice what is here right now – your feelings, thoughts, sounds, etc. Do not analyse or get caught up in them. Simply acknowledge their presence without judgement.

- **2nd minute – Focusing on the breath**: Shift your awareness to your breathing. Pay attention to your in-breath and out-breath. Choose one spot to focus on, e.g. the rising and falling of your abdomen, the sensation of air entering and leaving your nostrils, etc.

- **3rd minute – Expanding awareness to the entire body**: Bring your attention to your body-as-a-whole. One way to do this is to envision your in-breath travelling to all parts of your body. Notice physical sensations, e.g. your back leaning against the chair, your feet in contact with the ground, etc.

- As with all the other mindfulness practices, if you notice your mind ruminating anytime during this experience, gently acknowledge it and return your focus to the *here and now*.

- When the time is up, slowly open your eyes if they were closed. Bring your awareness back to the room and get on with your day.

Tip

Let go of the idea of "success", "failure" or "emptying the mind" when you are practising mindfulness. There is no such thing as a "perfect way" of doing it. The only discipline involved is regular and frequent practice. Thus, go through it with an attitude of openness, curiosity and kindness to yourself.

Chapter Summary & Homework

Mindfulness is the practice of bringing our awareness to the present moment in a non-judgemental manner. Focusing on the *here and now* helps manage rumination and prevents the downward spiral of negative thoughts and emotions.

While we cannot stop thoughts from surfacing, we can change the way we relate to them by using an observer's mind. In so-doing, we start to embrace our thoughts as passing mental events instead of treating all of them as facts.

Several mindfulness practices are recommended in this chapter. You may take to some more than the others. Experiment how you can incorporate into your daily routine those practices that work better for you. Slowly ease into making mindfulness part of your lifestyle.

Try This!

1. Use your observer's mind to notice some of the thoughts that popped up today. Were the emotions associated with those thoughts more or less intense compared to how you would normally treat them?

2. In the upcoming week, select one activity in your daily routine (e.g. washing up, eating, doing chores, etc.) and do it with an attitude of mindfulness. After completing it, reflect on the following questions in a curious, non-judgmental manner:

    a. What did you notice during the process?

    b. How is this different from the way you normally go about this activity?

3. Find a conducive time and location to practice the 3-minute breathing space. If you prefer, you may search for audio guides on the internet. After that, reflect on the following questions in a curious, non-judgmental manner:

    a. What did you notice during the process?

4. How is this different from the way you normally relate to your thoughts, feelings or body?

5. Many people may have some challenge starting a
    new habit like mindfulness. What are some possible
    obstacles for you in implementing this?

6. Go through the lists of mindfulness practices in this
    chapter and select those which you want to
    implement as part of your personal DEMS plan (in
    chapter 6).

5
S: Sleep

Sleep and emotional health often go hand in hand. Solid, restorative sleep energizes our minds and bodies, while poor sleep does the opposite.

Seth J. Gillihan

When Carl's low moods became overwhelming, his sleep patterns got interrupted. While he wanted to sleep, his mind was flooded with memories of his marriage as he laid on his bed. He thought about the happy times and the challenging times. Then came the remorse and regrets. This could go on for an hour or two, even though he was already physically and mentally exhausted. His rumination about his marriage soon became replaced by anxieties about having insomnia. The more he worried about not being able to sleep, the more he was kept awake.

It is common for people going through a difficult time to have some trouble sleeping. You could be faced with having too little sleep, or too much of it. Both can be detrimental to your personal well-being.

Too little sleep: A nervous system that is on high alert, which is typical after a traumatic or distressing event, can affect your ability to wind down. You might find yourself having intense thoughts and emotions while trying to rest. Insomnia – difficulties in falling asleep, staying asleep or going back to bed after you wake up in the middle of the night – can become an issue. Apart from social withdrawal and heightened feelings of loneliness, insufficient sleep can also lead to a weakened immunity, irritability, tiredness and trouble concentrating during the day.

Too much sleep: Having too much of sleep is not necessarily a good thing. Compared to having insufficient sleep, oversleeping affects a lesser percentage of people. Nevertheless, its impact is similar. You might find it more difficult to control your thoughts and emotions. As a result of having too little or too much sleep, the lowered levels of body and mental energy might, in turn, cause your low moods, anxieties and stress to escalate, creating a downward spiral.

Just about right: To enhance your well-being, it is important to have sufficient sleep. The amount of sleep you need depends on your age – newborns spend most of the day sleeping, while elderly people typically require less sleep compared to their younger days. Just as how our bodies need air, food and water, adults require between 6 to 9 hours of shut eye each night for optimal well-being.

Just to note – I use "night" to refer to the sleeping period as that is the norm for most people. Because of shift work or other circumstances, some of you may sleep in the day instead. The principles shared in this chapter can also be adapted to your situation.

> **Remember**
>
> Ample rest feeds you with energy to manage psychological flooding more effectively. Your mind will be able to notice the onslaught of thoughts without getting caught up in them, and mindfully shift your awareness away (read about *mindfulness* in Chapter 4 if you haven't already done so).

In the subsequent sections, I discuss some ways which people have used to manage sleep problems, with an emphasis on insomnia. This will be followed by a recent development in how mindfulness can help you sleep.

Pathways to Healthy Sleep

A rising concern, studies have found that insomnia affects about a third of the population in the US and UK. People are looking for solutions to their sleep problems. Try searching about insomnia on the internet and you will get tonnes of results showing you the many different ways to help you achiever healthier sleep. Common advice include:

Refraining from caffeine. Many who struggle with insomnia might resort to caffeine to help them combat the daytime tiredness. Doing so might, in turn, perpetuate the insomnia. Found in teas, coffees and some other beverages, caffeine promotes alertness and can remain in your body for six hours or more. Thus, it is commonly advised to refrain from caffein past noon to ensure that it does not keep you from falling sleepy at night.

Building sleep drive. Your body possesses a sleep drive which tells you that it's time for bed. From the time you get up and about in the morning, your sleep drive grows by the hour, causing to become more tired as the day progresses. A strong sleep drive helps you to sleep longer and more deeply at night. Studies found that taking naps, especially late in the day, reduces your sleep drive and disrupts your ability to sleep well at night. Besides avoiding naps, waking up at around the same time each day and keeping physically and mentally active during the day can boost your sleep drive. This alludes to the importance of incorporating engaging activities such as exercises, work and leisure (see Chapter 3) into your daily routine.

Having a conducive pre-sleep routine. Start letting your mind and body wind down about an hour before your bedtime. During this period, you should perform more relaxing activities such as light reading, listening to soothing music, simple stretches, brushing your teeth or getting dressed for bed. A warm bath an hour or so before bedtime can help you fall asleep faster as your core temperature drops after you come out of the shower. Drinking a glass of warm water achieves the same effect. The gradual cooling of your body augments your circadian rhythm, or sleep-wake cycle, signalling to your brain that it is night time (cooler temperatures compared to the day). Where possible, you might want to refrain from stimulating activities such as watching TV, doing work, exercising or playing computer games during this time.

Having a dimmed or dark room. Darkness matters for good sleep. Lights inhibits the production of melatonin – the "sleep hormone" responsible for helping you feel relax and drowsy. The absence of light signals to the body that it is time to rest. In line with circadian rhythm, dimming the lights before bedtime prepares your mind and body for sleep. Consider installing dimmer switches or warmer lights around the house. Dimmed and warm lights also exude feelings of calmness and relaxation. Conversely, the lights emitted from screens, whether TV, mobile devices or computers, can disrupt your circadian rhythm and should be minimised before bedtime. While sleeping, it is advised to keep the room dark. Blackout curtains can be used to block lights entering through the windows. Some people also find wearing eye masks to bed helpful. If a night light is required, consider using one with a red bulb – the wavelength of red light is less disruptive to sleep compared to the rest.

Using the room only for sleep: If you have been doing work-related tasks in your bedroom, such as typing emails or reports, your brain might associate the room with work or productivity. Similarly, if you play computer or mobile games in the room, your brain and body might subconsciously associate it with leisure. These associations could make it harder for you to fall asleep at night. If you have no choice but to work from your bedroom, you could try mitigating these associations by setting certain boundaries between work and sleep. For instance, you could make your bed when you wake up in the morning, and not sit or lay on it during work hours. You could also put a partition or a book shelf to segregate your bed from your working space. These can signal to your brain whether you are in your work mode or resting mode.

Drinking less water before bedtime: It is not uncommon for people with insomnia to wake up in the middle of the night to use the bathroom, only to find it difficult to fall back to sleep. Hydration is important, as you've learnt in Chapter 2. So, ensure you meet your water intake requirements for the day. But cut down on drinking about an hour or so before bedtime and empty your bladder just before you go to bed. This minimises the chances of you getting up to go to the toilet at night.

Sleep, Anxiety and Avoidance Behaviours

It is important to understand that sleep occurs in four or five cycles of different depths and types throughout the night, e.g. light sleep, deep sleep, REM (rapid eye movement) sleep. From being awake, it usually takes about 10 to 20 minutes for your brain waves to slow down before drifting to sleep. Deep sleep usually happens in the first two cycles, while REM sleep in the late night and wee hours of the morning. Around 50 per cent of our sleep comprise of light sleep. Typically, each cycle lasts about 90 minutes. You may or may not notice a slight awakening time between each cycle. That's when you get up to flip over to the other side or go to the bathroom. That's part and parcel of our sleep. Remember – no one is able to sleep continuously throughout the night.

Tips

If you are keen to track the quality of your sleep, some smart watches and fitness watches are able to measure the amount of sleep you have in the various cycles.

While most people are able to fall asleep at bedtime and drift back to sleep after the brief waking periods between cycles, you might find it a challenge if there is psychological flooding. Thinking that it is insomnia that has kept you up, your mind might be filled with thoughts about not being able to fall back to sleep or the consequences of insufficient rest. Being in this state can be distressing, anxiety-provoking and even fear-inducing. As a result of these thoughts and emotions, you might be kept wide awake. If this goes on over the course of weeks and months, your mind might become conditioned anticipate being wakeful and anxious during bedtime, even though that's not what you want!

In attempting to deal with this state of wakefulness, some of you might have tried things like getting out of bed to have a drink, take a bath, watch TV or pop a pill. Psychologists found that while these might sometimes work, they can also become "avoidance behaviours" – actions you adopt to avoid insomnia. Avoidance behaviours perpetuate the maintenance cycle of insomnia as they feed on your anxieties of not being able to sleep, and in turn keep you awake. I know. It's not pretty. But that's how anxiety works – when you try to control it, there's a chance it might get worse.

Remember

Tired, frustrated, angry and worried – all these emotions trigger a feeling of being in danger and further feed wakefulness; they're the stuff that insomnia thrives upon.

- Elaine Foreman and Clair Pollard

Using Mindfulness to Improve Insomnia

Instead of turning to avoidance behaviours, recent research found promising outcomes in using mindfulness as a response to insomnia. You see, people who sleep well don't really "try hard" to fall asleep – they just get on with their day normally and doze off during bedtime. But if you are going through depression, anxieties or stress, your mind might be psychologically flooded with worries and thinking up ways to fix your insomnia. Mindfulness helps you take a step back from your thoughts, giving your mind and body some respite and detachment from the worries.

Mindfulness During the Day

Practising mindfulness during the day is a good exercise in training your observer's mind and conditioning your mind to relate to your thoughts differently. There is less pressure to combat insomnia during daytime, making the practise of mindfulness more about a personal discipline rather than a solution for sleep.

A selection of simple *mindfulness practices* can be found in Chapter 4. Doing these exercises regularly helps you to be more adept in shifting your focus from your thoughts to the present moment experiences. This can come in handy when the notice the onset of psychological flooding as you are lying on your bed at night. You will not just experience the benefits during or immediately after the mindfulness practices. The positive effects endure long after the practices have ended.

Mindful Resting at Night

When faced with wakefulness while you are lying on your bed at night, give the following **mindful resting** exercise a go! Give yourself between 10 to 15 minutes to go through the various segments. As you do this, remind yourself that the aim of practising mindfulness is not to get you to fall asleep, although sleep might come as a by-product. Mindfulness produces a state of mind in you that makes falling asleep more likely.

1. Start by recognising the thoughts and emotions that are already present in your mind and body. Acknowledge them non-judgementally, and gently remind yourself that you do not need to analyse them. Like an observer, notice these thoughts and emotions without reacting to them (e.g. "Oh, I'm having this thought about insomnia again", or "Hmm. I notice I'm having these worries about...").

2. Next, shift your awareness from your thoughts to your bodily sensations. Notice how your body feels lying on the mattress. Pay attention how the muscles in your arms, back and legs are feeling. Pick up the temperature of the air and the sensations of your clothing on your skin.

3. Next, allow the surrounding sounds to flow into your ears. Focus on the quality of each sound. Is it loud or soft? Is it near or far? Is it coming or going? Is it low pitched or high pitched? Does it repeat? If you notice any thoughts arise, simply acknowledge them

before gently shifting your awareness back to the
sounds.

4. Finally, shift your attention to your breathing. Pay
    attention to your in-breath and out-breath.
    Concentrate on one spot at a time, e.g. the rising and
    falling of your abdomen, the sensation of air
    entering and leaving your nostrils, etc.

If you find yourself dozing off briefly during this
mindfulness exercise, acknowledge that too. Should sleep
arrive, welcome it. If it doesn't, don't fret about it. And
you will learn why in the next section.

A Sense of Acceptance

By now, you already know that if you fret or worry over
not being able to fall asleep, your mind gets more
stimulated, making sleep more elusive than it was. Apart
from that, another subtle thing that could happen is that
your brain might perceive insomnia as a threat. The
avoidance behaviours and anxious ruminations signal to
your brain that insomnia is a powerful enemy which you
desperately need to evade from. As with any threat or
danger, we become more vigilant, guarded and alert. Alas,
it becomes harder to wind down and relax.

However, with mindfulness, you begin to relate to
insomnia differently. Instead of actively resisting or
fighting insomnia, you adopt a posture of acceptance. By
acceptance, I do not mean resigning yourself to the
situation or feeling hopeless about it. Here, "acceptance"

is defined as your personal, active decision to allow the unpleasant experiences exist without trying to dismiss or fix them. You don't run away from insomnia or try to fight it – you treat it non-judgementally, as you would with the thoughts that pop into your mind when doing the mindfulness practices. If sleep still evades you, Foreman and Pollard (2016) suggest that lying in bed without resisting wakefulness can also provide some rest, and that the key to sleeping is having an "accepting and relaxed attitude to being awake at night".

Accepting insomnia and the thoughts and emotions associated with it can be an important step in your journey towards healthier sleep. You are, in fact, sending a signal to your brain that insomnia is no longer a danger or an enemy. This neutralises the threat that was once posed to you mind when you were fighting it. When you face and accept the very thing you are feeling anxious or fearful about, it loses its power over you.

Handles to Manage Oversleeping

Oversleeping affects a considerably lesser proportion of the population compared to insomnia. Like insomnia, it can also contribute to fatigue and mood problems. Here're some strategies you can adopt to manage oversleeping:

- **Go to bed at the same time every night**: Have a fixed bedtime and waking-up time contributes to healthier sleep. This applies to both weekdays and weekends! Sometimes, the inability to fall asleep during bedtime throws your circadian rhythm off and can inadvertently result in oversleeping. To address this, refer to the principles and tips in the sections on *pathways to healthy sleep* and *using mindfulness to improve insomnia.*

- **Allow sunlight to penetrate your room in the morning**: Just as how darkness makes it easier to sleep, sunlight sends a message to your body that it's time to wake up. Consider leaving an opening in the curtains or blinds to allow the morning light to shine in. Alternatively, you can also consider one of those wake-up light alarm clocks that simulates the sunrise. Where possible, time the lights to grow progressively brighter 20 to 40 minutes before the alarm goes off.

- **Schedule activities in the morning**: You could be tempted to isolate yourself as a result of your depression and anxieties. Social withdrawal, coupled with the lack of energy and motivation, could mean more time spent in bed. In the previous chapters, we've talked about how such forms of withdrawal can create a downward spiral in your moods. If you're not up to it to meet people, you could schedule activities such as making breakfast, running an errand, reading a book or taking a walk in the morning. Plan these activities in advance. These could give you more impetus to get out of bed. When the moods are not so overwhelming, consider arranging breakfast with friends or family, or to taking a stroll with someone.

Oversleeping can also be in indication of underlying medical conditions such as sleep apnoea and hypothyroidism. Consulting a doctor will get your symptoms assessed and treated accordingly.

Chapter Summary & Homework

In this chapter, we learnt how sufficient sleep (7 to 9 hours for adults) provides you with body and mental energy to manage psychological flooding more effectively. Conversely, insufficient sleep can affect your moods and functioning during the day. The following can help you achieve healthier sleep:

- Refraining from caffeine.

- Building sleep drive.

- Having a conducive pre-sleep routine.

- Having a dimmed or dark room.

- Using the room only for sleep.

Sometimes, trying hard to fall asleep can be counter-productive. Fretting over insomnia causes your mind to treat it as a threat and be further stimulated. In turn, you can be kept awake. The attitude of non-judgement and acceptance that mindfulness brings helps neutralise this sense of threat, creating a more conducive condition to welcome sleep. Even if sleep doesn't show up, lying on your bed peacefully can be restful, and preferrable to battling insomnia.

Try This!

1. How would you describe your sleep in general? Do
    you experience difficulty falling asleep and/or
    staying asleep?

2. How do you know if you have adequate or
    inadequate rest?

3. What is your usual routine in the two hours leading to your bedtime?

4. Are you currently using any avoidance behaviours in order to sleep? What might they be? To what extent have they been helpful?

5. If you could, what would you like to change about
    your sleep?

6. In the upcoming week, choose a night to practise
    mindful resting before you sleep (see section
    "Mindfulness at night").

7. Go through the lists of strategies and tips in this
    chapter, and select those which you want to
    implement as part of your personal DEMS plan.

6
Your Personal DEMS Plan

If you fail to plan,
you plan to fail.

Benjamin Franklin

Wow… you've almost come to the end of the book! Hopefully you have gleaned some insights into how diet, engaging activities, mindfulness and sleep can help enhance your personal well-being and keep psychological flooding at bay. To recap, here's a summary of the four pillars of DEMS.

Diet: To provide your body & mind with the energy they need to keep psychological flooding at bay, ensure that your diet includes i) Regular, balanced meals, ii) mood-boosting foods and iii) ample hydration.

Engaging activities – Schedule into your daily & weekly routine activities that engage & energise your mind. This includes i) work, ii) exercise and iii) leisure activities. Increasing the number of nourishing activities or pairing draining activities with nourishing ones can be mood-lifting.

Mindfulness – Find regular pockets of time during the week for mindfulness practices. Mindfulness helps manage rumination and prevents the downward spiral of negative thoughts and emotions. While you cannot stop thoughts from surfacing, you can change the way you relate to them by using an observer's mind and practising non-judgement.

Sleep – Adjust lifestyle and sleep hygiene so as to achieve better quality and quantity of sleep. Sufficient sleep (7 to 9 hours) provides you with the body and mental energy required to manage psychological flooding more effectively.

Besides reading through the previous chapters, I also hope that you have had the opportunity to do the homework ("Try This!"). You will now draw upon the learning that emerged from your reading and homework to design your personal DEMS plan. This is the plan that you will put in place to make DEMS an integral part of your lifestyle moving forward. I'm not just talking about the week ahead. As with any new habit, it will take a few months for DEMS to become more naturally assimilated into your regular routine. Effort is also needed to sustain it for the years to come.

During the initial period, your DEMS lifestyle will take some getting used to. You might even feel some resistance. That's expected. We're talking about overriding some of your existing habitual behaviours, and making new changes with deliberate control. So, hang in there and press on. Even when the going gets tough.

I will keep this chapter short so that you can spend some time planning. There is also no chapter summary at the end. As for homework, you have only one for this final chapter – that is, to complete your personal DEMS plan.

In the following pages, you will see the personal DEMS plan which I give to my clients and coachees to fill up. Brief explanations of each component of the DEMS plan will provided in the next section. Feel free to replicate this template in your notebook or computer document for your personal use. You can even customise the sections and format to something that suits your preference – as long as it works for you. If you would like a soft copy of the template, feel free to email your request to *approach.justin@gmail.com*. I'd be more than happy to send it to you.

DEMS Template

MY LONG-TERM GOAL	
D: DIET	
ACTION STEPS	FREQUENCY
POTENTIAL BARRIERS	POSSIBLE SOLUTIONS

E: ENGAGING ACTIVITIES	
ACTION STEPS	FREQUENCY
POTENTIAL BARRIERS	POSSIBLE SOLUTIONS
ACTION STEPS	FREQUENCY

M: MINDFULNESS	
ACTION STEPS	FREQUENCY
POTENTIAL BARRIERS	POSSIBLE SOLUTIONS
ACTION STEPS	FREQUENCY

S: SLEEP	
ACTION STEPS	FREQUENCY
POTENTIAL BARRIERS	POSSIBLE SOLUTIONS
TO BE REVIEWED ON:	

Components of Personal DEMS Plan

1. Long-term goal

The first step in designing your DEMS plan is to define your long-term goal. You can describe in one to three sentences how you would like your mental and emotional well-being to be two years from today. You may refer to the homework in Chapter 1 (Try This! - Item 1) for inspiration. You may also use the SMART goal technique to craft your goal. A SMART goal is one that is:

- Specific

- Measurable

- Attainable

- Relevant

- Time-bound

Here're some examples of long-term goals:

"It is [future date] and I can better manage my emotions. Regardless of how my marriage turns out, I will feel at peace knowing I have done my best. I feel healthy and energised because of the positive changes I have made to my lifestyle." - Carl

"It is [future date]. My anxiety score has lowered to the normal range. I no longer suffer from panic attacks, and I can notice when unhelpful or distorted thoughts are popping up in my mind." - Pam

"By [future date], I will achieve a better work-life balance. With the inclusion of nourishing activities and the regular practice of mindfulness, I will be able to handle work stress more effectively. My relationship with my family will also improve, and we will spend more quality time together during the week." - Keith

Remember

Begin with the end in mind.

- Stephen Covey

2. My action steps & frequency

After defining your long-term goal, you will then list down the concrete steps you have to take for D, E, M and S respectively in order to work towards your goal. Your action steps will comprise of tasks you need to do, new habits you want to adopt and changes you want to make to your regular routine from today.

You will also indicate the frequency which you will carry out each step: daily, weekly, fortnightly, monthly, ad-hoc, etc. Go through the principles, strategies, tips and homework in chapters 2 to 5, and customise an action plan that you think might work for your particular life situation and context.

These action steps can evolve and be modified along the way. It is not cast in stone. For the initial period, I recommend you take achievable "baby steps" rather than putting in place a challenging task. It's like driving – you start slowly with the first gear, and gradually shift to higher gears as the car picks up speed. The rationale is to set yourself up for small successes rather than being deflated over a plan which you have difficulty accomplishing. In this regard, you may want to start by having no more than four action steps for each component of DEMS instead of a crafting long list that might be too overwhelming.

Here's an example how Pam's action steps for *Engaging Activities* changed over the months.

Month 1-3:

Action Steps for "E"	Frequency
Take a 10-minute walk around the park.	Once a week
Bake cakes for friends and family.	Once a month

Month 4-6:

Action Steps for "E"	Frequency
Take a 20-minute walk around the neighbourhood park.	Two or three times a week

Baking and exploring new recipes.	Twice a month
Do simple, light stretches after waking up.	On weekends

Keith also modified his actions steps as he gained momentum. Here's how his *mindfulness* plan evolved:

Month 1-2:

Action Steps for "M"	Frequency
Do a mindful body scan before going to bed.	Once a week
Do mindful breathing (1-minute) while taking breaks at work	Daily

Month 3-6:

Action Steps for "M"	Frequency
Do the 3-minute breathing space.	At least once a week

Do mindful breathing (1-minute) when I start to feel stressed.	Daily
Do a mindful walk in nature with family.	Once a month.
Read a book on mindfulness.	Ad-hoc

While the examples above showed how the action steps increased in variety and frequency over time, it is also plausible for the opposite to happen – that is, for you to cut back on the intensity and regularity. And that's perfectly fine as well. This could happen for various reasons. For instance, you might have planned something a little more challenging that what you can manage. Or you could run into certain circumstances or barriers that affect your progress.

Remember

Do something today that your future self will thank you for.

- Sean Patrick Flanery

The secret of getting ahead is getting started.

- Sally Berger

3. Potential barriers and possible solutions

When implementing your DEMS plan, it is possible that obstacles and challenges will arise. External barriers could be things like the lack of resources, support or time. There might also be internal barriers such as the lack of motivation, knowledge or confidence. Here, you will brainstorm and list down what these barriers might be. Come up with one or two barriers for D, E, M and S respectively. And try doing so in a mindful, non-judgemental manner instead of being led away by worry or stress.

After identifying the barriers, brainstorm one or two ways to overcome each challenge. You could also talk to your family and friends to get some ideas on possible solutions.

Remember

If you can find a path with no obstacles, it probably doesn't lead anywhere.

- Frank A. Clark

4. Review date

Set a date to review your implementation of DEMS. Start with a fortnightly review, followed by a monthly review once you begin getting used to the routine. Regular reviews (at least once a month) will help you keep track of your progress. Keep an open mind, and allow some flexibility to make modifications to your original plan as you review. Here are some review questions you can use:

- What are some key highlights of my DEMS journey so far?

- What has been working well for me?

- What has been challenging?

- What changes can I make to my personal DEMS plan so it can be more relevant / achievable / impactful / meaningful?

- Who (or what) can help me in implementing DEMS more effectively? How?

Remember

It is good to have an end to journey toward; but it is the journey that matters, in the end.

- Ursula K. Le Guin

A final word

Difficult times will always happen. Life is unlikely to be smooth sailing all the time. Recovery from mental and emotional health problems can sometimes be a bumpy process. And in case this point was not made clear in the previous chapters, DEMS is not a magical pill that makes your problems disappear. Instead, DEMS is a form of prioritising your personal welling by adjusting your diet, scheduling engaging activities, practising mindfulness and having ample sleep…. so that when the going gets tough, you are less likely to enter into the downward spiral brought about by depression, anxiety and stress.

My hope for you is this: As DEMS becomes a habitual part of your lifestyle, you will attain a healthier level of mind – one that will enable you to notice the onset of psychological flooding, curb ruminations and relate to your thoughts in a non-judgemental manner. In so-doing, you are overriding some of your old, unhelpful ways of thinking and behaving.

Here's to many healthy journeys ahead.

References

Foreman, Elaine I., and Pollard, Clair. (2016) *Cognitive Behavioural Therapy*. Icon Books.

Gillihan, Seth J. (2018) *Cognitive Behavioural Therapy Made Simple*. Althea Press.

Ilardi, Stephen. (2010) *The Depression Cure: The 6-Step Program to Beat Depression without Drugs*. Da Capo Lifelong Books.

Rowe, Sara Milne. (2018) *The SHED Method*. Penguin Books.

www.ingramcontent.com/pod-product-compliance
Lightning Source LLC
Chambersburg PA
CBHW061350250726